Yusuf Rushdi

Patent Foramen Ovale

Yusuf Rushdi

Patent Foramen Ovale

LAP LAMBERT Academic Publishing

Impressum / Imprint

Bibliografische Information der Deutschen Nationalbibliothek: Die Deutsche Nationalbibliothek verzeichnet diese Publikation in der Deutschen Nationalbibliografie; detaillierte bibliografische Daten sind im Internet über http://dnb.d-nb.de abrufbar.

Alle in diesem Buch genannten Marken und Produktnamen unterliegen warenzeichen-, marken- oder patentrechtlichem Schutz bzw. sind Warenzeichen oder eingetragene Warenzeichen der jeweiligen Inhaber. Die Wiedergabe von Marken, Produktnamen, Gebrauchsnamen, Handelsnamen, Warenbezeichnungen u.s.w. in diesem Werk berechtigt auch ohne besondere Kennzeichnung nicht zu der Annahme, dass solche Namen im Sinne der Warenzeichen- und Markenschutzgesetzgebung als frei zu betrachten wären und daher von jedermann benutzt werden dürften.

Bibliographic information published by the Deutsche Nationalbibliothek: The Deutsche Nationalbibliothek lists this publication in the Deutsche Nationalbibliografie; detailed bibliographic data are available in the Internet at http://dnb.d-nb.de.

Any brand names and product names mentioned in this book are subject to trademark, brand or patent protection and are trademarks or registered trademarks of their respective holders. The use of brand names, product names, common names, trade names, product descriptions etc. even without a particular marking in this work is in no way to be construed to mean that such names may be regarded as unrestricted in respect of trademark and brand protection legislation and could thus be used by anyone.

Coverbild / Cover image: www.ingimage.com

Verlag / Publisher:
LAP LAMBERT Academic Publishing
ist ein Imprint der / is a trademark of
OmniScriptum GmbH & Co. KG
Bahnhofstraße 28, 66111 Saarbrücken, Deutschland / Germany
Email: info@lap-publishing.com

Herstellung: siehe letzte Seite /
Printed at: see last page
ISBN: 978-3-659-83269-7

Zugl. / Approved by: London, Queen Mary University of London, 2006

Copyright © 2016 OmniScriptum GmbH & Co. KG
Alle Rechte vorbehalten. / All rights reserved. Saarbrücken 2016

Dedication

To my parents, wife, daughter, siblings and in-laws.

I thank you all for being there for me and for your continuous encouragement and support.

All would not have been possible without the spiritual hand of the most gracious and the most powerful, God almighty.

Table of Contents

Abbreviations 4
Abstract 5
Aim 7
Introduction 8
Materials and Methods 12
   Selection of Subjects 13
      The retrospective study 13
      The prospective study 14
   Diagnostic Criteria 14
      Questionnaire 15
   Inclusion Criteria 18
   Exclusion Criteria 19
   Variables of Interest 19
Objectives of the Study 20
Transcranial Doppler Protocol [39] 21
Results 27
   Retrospective study 27
   Prospective study results 44
   The format of the report 45
Discussion 52
Conclusions 55
Future Proposals 56
REFERENCES 57

List of Figures

Figure 1 Locating the middle cerebral artery using acoustic coupling medium and an ultrasound probe to locate the artery. 23
Figure 2 Locating the middle cerebral artery and making sure the signals stay stable during VM or coughing. 23
Figure 3 Agitated saline pushed back and forth vigorously between the two 10ml syringes about 10 times. Visible air should not be injected. 24
Figure 4 Transcranial Doppler shunt study recording the middle cerebral artery flow through the skull before intravenous microbubbles injection. 24
Figure 5 Transcranial Doppler readings of middle cerebral artery during the valsalva manoeuvre. Reading kept stable for the procedure to proceed. 25

List of Tables

Table 1 Gender ... 27
Table 2 Statistics ... 27
Table 3 Occupation ... 28
Table 4 Location of arterial embolism / pain ... 29
Table 5 Onset of symptoms ... 30
Table 6 Duration of complaints ... 30
Table 7 Frequency of symptoms ... 30
Table 8 Cause of embolus ... 31
Table 9 Immobilisation ... 31
Table 10 Pregnancy ... 32
Table 11 Recent Surgery ... 32
Table 12 Hypercoaguble state ... 32
Table 13 Previous DVT ... 33
Table 14 Other Predisposing factors of a DVT ... 33
Table 15 Congenital abnormalities ... 34
Table 16 Neurological procedures ... 34
Table 17 Bleeding disorders ... 35
Table 18 Liver disease ... 35
Table 19 Previous stroke ... 35
Table 20 Diabetes Mellitus ... 36
Table 21 Other past medical histories ... 36
Table 22 Smoking ... 37
Table 23 Frequency of smoking ... 38
Table 24 Alcohol consumption ... 39
Table 25 Frequency of Alcohol consumption ... 39
Table 26 Family history ... 40
Table 27 Positive signs ... 40
Table 28 Hypercoagulable state screening ... 40
Table 29 Ruling out DVT ... 41
Table 30 Time duration of DVT screening ... 41
Table 31 Imagining techniques ... 42
Table 32 Treatment modalities ... 43
Table 33 Mortality ... 43
Table 34 Agitated saline testing ... 44

Abbreviations

ASD	Atrial Septal Defect
ASA	Atrial Septal Aneurysm
CVA	Cerebro Vascular Accident
c-TOE	contrast- Transoesophageal echocardiography
c-TCD	contrast- Trancranial Doppler
CT	Computerized Tomography
DOB	Date of Birth
DOA	Date of Admission
DOD	Date of Discharge
DVT	Deep Vein Thrombosis
DM	Diabetes Mellitus
ECHO	Echocardiogram
ECG	Electrocardiography
LCH	London Chest Hospital
LA	Left Atrium
MCA	Middle Cerebral Artery
MRI	Magnetic Resonance Imaging
MA	Migraine with Aura
OSAS	Obstructive Sleep Apnoea Syndrome
PFO	Patent Foramen Ovale
RA	Right Atrium
RLS	Right to Left Shunt
RLH	Royal London Hospital
SPSS	Statistical and Presentational System Software.
SPAC	Stroke Prevention: Assessment of risk in a Community
SBH	St. Bartholomew's Hospital
TOF	Tetrology of Fallot
TOE	Transoesophageal echocardiography
TTE	Transthoracic echocardiography
TCD	Trancranial Doppler
U/S	Ultra Sound
VM	Valsalva Manoeuvre
VSD	Ventricular septal defect

Abstract

Introduction:

Peripheral arterial embolus carries a high mortality, related to the underlying disease rather than to the effects of the embolus itself. Recently, with the advent of transthoracic echo techniques, it has been suggested that up to 25% of the population have a previously undiagnosed patent foramen ovale, which would allow clot from the venous circulation to enter the arterial tree and cause an arterial embolus. The aim of this study was to examine a cohort of patients who had suffered an arterial embolus to see whether a PFO was identifiable.

Methods:

An audit of ten years of records from the Royal London Hospital, London Chest Hospital and the St. Bartholomew's was conducted. This study was in two parts; a retrospective part involving a notes audit and a prospective study on selected patients from that audit. Data and relevant information on patients with peripheral vascular disease was collected into a structured questionnaire addressing presenting and past complaints, examination and treatment. Patients with peripheral arterial embolism were identified. Out of 71 patients with arterial embolism 15 patients were found in which a right to left shunt (patent foramen ovale) was suspected and 3 of them had already had a PFO closure. To identify a right-to-left shunt in the 12 patients identified as requiring prospective study, an agitated saline test with Transcranial Doppler ultrasound with valsalva manoeuvre was carried out on 5, the remaining 7 patients being unavailable for follow-up.

Results:

The retrospective study on the 71 patients revealed a high male prevalence, 75% with predisposing factors to DVT, about 70% being smokers and unfortunately 85% with no documented cause of their symptoms, though 84.4% of patients had a significant past history of vascular symptoms.

In this small study, none of the patients tested from the prospective study were found to have evidence of a right to left shunt. All of the patients had some sort of predisposing factor such as DVT. However, of selected 15 patients, 3 had already had a percutaneous PFO closure.

Conclusions:

It was not possible to identify and study enough patients in this retrospective study to be sure, but it seems that the incidence of a right to left shunt in the study group is no higher than that found in the general population (3/15, 20%). There was a high prevalence of male smokers in the paradoxical embolus group with associated predisposing factors leading to a DVT.

Aim

The aim of this small retrospective-prospective study was to try and identify patients with a paradoxical arterial embolism associated with Patent Foramen Ovale (PFO) or other right to left shunt.

The hypothesis of the study was that when a PFO is found with a peripheral arterial embolism it increases the risk of a DVT causing an arterial embolism and that paradoxical embolus may account for a higher number of acute arterial emboli than has been recognised previously.

Peripheral Arterial Embolism and its Relationship to Patent Foramen Ovale

Introduction

Patent foramen ovale is an interatrial communication known since the time of Galen[2, 4]. In 1564 Botallo described the presence of a PFO at birth[1, 2, 4]. Some still refer to a PFO as the Foramen of Botallo[2, 4]. In 1877 Cornheim described a paradoxical embolus related to a PFO[2, 4]. Patients with PFO have no characteristic physical or electro-cardio graphic findings[4]. Some may present with a history of stroke or a transient ischemic event of undefined aetiology[2, 4].

The foramen ovale is a slit-like opening in the atrial septum at the site of the foramen secundum of the septum primum. In intrauterine life, the foramen ovale has the important role of transmitting highly oxygenated inferior vena caval blood to the left atrium. High right atrial (RA) pressure in the fetus keeps the valve of the foramen ovale open. The left atrial pressure rises shortly after birth and the flap is lightly pressed against the septum secundum and closes the foramen ovale functionally[4]. Patency of the foramen ovale (PFO) has been identified as a potential risk factor for paradoxical embolism potentially followed by cerebral or peripheral ischemic events[3].

Although the underlying mechanism by which PFO accounts for the phenomenon is not entirely clear, the trans-septal passage of emboli from the right to the left sided chambers of the heart appear to play an important role [3, 30]. Moreover, 4.2% of patients with a documented PFO and previous embolism are at increased risk of recurrent thromboembolic events even under therapeutic anticoagulation[3]. Hoffman et al suggested that anatomic patency may persist for several months after birth and 50% of all infants have a probe-patent PFO at the end of the first year of life [4], and although this figure falls with age, 30% of the adult population probably have a PFO.

PFO is a failure of progression of the normal developmental process unlike an atrial septal defect (ASD) which is the partial or total deficiency of the atrial septum itself [4].

Ordinarily, a left-to-right shunt will cause no problems, but a right-to-left shunt, if large enough, will cause a low arterial O_2 tension (hypoxia) and severely limited exercise capacity.

In divers there is a risk of paradoxical embolism of gas bubbles (passage of bubbles into the arterial circulation), which form in the majority of divers in the venous circulation during decompression. Blood can flow in both directions within intra-atrial shunts at various phases of the cardiac cycle and some experts feel that a large atrial septal defect or PFO is a contra-indication to diving.

The Valsalva manoeuvre, used by most divers to adjust the pressure in the tympanic cavity during descent and ascent, can increase venous atrial pressure to the point that it forces blood containing bubbles across the PFO into the arterial circulation. Thus the usual filtering process of the lung is by-passed.

The average size of a PFO increases from a mean of 3.4mm in the first decade to 5.8mm in the tenth decade of life[2, 3, 4]. The larger the degree of interatrial shunting, the greater the incidence of subsequent transient ischaemic attack or stroke[4, 2]. Depending on the criteria used for diagnosis and the technology used for cardiac assessment, the prevalence of PFO in the healthy population is approximately 20 to 25% [24, 25, 27]. On the basis of prevalence, we can estimate that approximately 60 - 70 million Americans have a PFO[27]. Thus the detection of a PFO during the evaluation of a patient with stroke is not a surprising finding and the frequency of PFO detection in these patients can be as high as 40 - 45% [1, 23, 27]. PFO is now detected in 10% to 15% of the normal population using contrast echocardiography. Autopsy studies in otherwise normal hearts have shown a higher (27%) prevalence of patent foramen ovale. The prevalence found in autopsies among stroke patient is even higher (40%) [4, 5, 6].

With increasing evidence that PFOs are the culprit in paradoxical embolic events, paradoxical embolism through a PFO should be strongly considered in young patient with cryptogenic stroke and the relative importance of PFO is being re-evaluated [2, 7, 11].

The clinical diagnosis of paradoxical embolism is almost always presumptive and is suspected in patients who have a venous thrombus, a right to left shunt and evidence of arterial embolism [14, 15].

A definite diagnosis of paradoxical embolism is established when a thrombus is seen traversing the shunt[14,15]. Deep venous thrombosis are found with variable success in patients suspected of paradoxical embolism, and prevalence of DVT range from 9.5% to 88% depending on the timing and methods used for diagnosis[14, 15].

It was documented in a recent investigation that the prevalence of RLF shunt was significantly higher in patients suffering from migraine with aura (MA) than in healthy controls and similar to that found in young patients with stroke[35,36,37].

Obstructive Sleep Apnoea Syndrome (OSAS) is not a rare condition in the general population; its prevalence ranges from 0.3 to 8.5%[31, 33, 34]. A recent study revealed that a right to left shunt can occur through a PFO in subjects with OSAS during periods of nocturnal apnoea if the apnoea length is longer than 17 seconds.[31,32].

Echocardiography is a necessary tool for the diagnosis of PFO, which can be diagnosed by either colour flow Doppler or intravenous agitated saline contrast study. This is performed after obtaining optimal visualization of the atrial septum using transthoracic or if necessary, trans-oesophageal echocardiography[2, 16].

A trans-oesophageal echo provides better visualisation of the atrial septum and is therefore more sensitive than trans-thoracic echo for detecting PFO[2, 17].

When PFO is suspected in a stroke patient, if the trans-thoracic studies are negative the patient should undergo a transoesophageal echo with injected radio-opaque contrast medium together with micro bubbles injected into an antecubital vein[2, 17].

Bilateral Transcranial Doppler ultrasound (TCD) can be used to assess a right-to-left shunt, by monitoring both middle cerebral arteries during normal ventilation and during valsalva manoeuvre according to the Consensus Meeting of the European Society of Neurology[35,38]. The technique used is described in detail in the protocol for agitated saline test later on.

Right to left shunting is graded in consensus by an experienced cardiologist and radiologist as follows: Grade 0, no contrast agent passed from the right to the left atrium; Grade-1, 3-9 micro-bubbles passed from the right to the left atrium; Grade 2 is 10–29 and Grade 3, greater than 30 microbubbles[28, 29]. In 76 healthy volunteers, a trans-thoracic echocardiographic study using a well established, agitated saline contrast technique found that the prevalence of right to left shunting through a PFO was 5% when subjects were at rest and 18% when subjects performed a valsalva manoeuvre [12].

In the SPARC (Stroke Prevention: Assessment of Risk in a Community) study, the prevalence of right to left shunting increased from 14% in subjects at rest to 23% with the performance of various manoeuvres (release of valsalva manoeuvre and cough), which increased the right atrial pressure by increasing venous return[13]. When it is merely an isolated incidental finding, an asymptomatic PFO does not require treatment.

When a PFO is found in association with an otherwise unexplained neurological event, there is general agreement that the patient should be treated with anticoagulation, and in some cases, that the PFO should be closed. Medical treatment consists of the administration of warfarin with or without aspirin to prevent stroke recurrence.

Surgical PFO closure using double continuous suture has resulted in no recurrence of neurological events during follow up of one to four years but it require thoracotomy and cardiopulmonary bypass[18-20].

Cardiac surgery is highly invasive and a much more satisfactory alternative involves insertion of a catheter-delivered closure device; this is an emerging option for the treatment of PFO. It requires twenty four to forty eight hours of hospital stay and aspirin or warfarin for six months post procedure[21-23].

Materials and Methods

The study is in a form of an audit where data was collected from the last ten years of patient records form the London Chest Hospital, Royal London Hospital and St. Bartholomew's Hospital.

The Clinical Effectiveness Unit carried out an initial search of records based on the term "paradoxical embolus" and this generated a list of about 900 patients. A refined search of these records using the search term "peripheral arterial embolism", generated a shorter list of about 450 records. Combining the search terms "RLS" and "Peripheral arterial embolism" cut the number of records down to 71, and 15 of these were thought likely to have a PFO, based on a filtering questionnaire applied to the notes, and which yielded important information on the epidemiology of peripheral arterial embolus. Out of the remaining 15 patients, three had already had a PFO closed using a percutaneous device.

The original 71 patients were analysed for epidemiological data on the aetiology of arterial embolus as a retrospective study.

Of the 15 patients selected from the original 71, thought to have a PFO, the twelve who had not had a closure device fitted were invited to attend an outpatients clinic for an agitated saline test. Ethics committee approval for this mildly invasive test was not sought since it is now a recognised part of the diagnostic armamentarium for this disease. In the event only five patients could be traced and studied. This became the prospective side of the study.

Selection of Subjects

- Data Source

The retrospective study

This included the collection of data on 71 patients seen in the hospitals over a ten year period on a questionnaire in the context of demography, presenting and past complaints, investigations performed and treatment modalities from the records of selected hospitals (RLH, SBH, LCH).

Patients with arterial emboli were identified using the headline diagnosis given on the hospital computer database. Medical records were obtained and were then studied in more detail using a notes questionnaire which asked the following questions:

1. The main presenting complaint, particularly concentrating on peripheral arterial embolus or stroke
2. Profession
3. Chronology of onset of symptoms
4. Course of the disease
5. Whether there was a predisposing factor for DVT such as immobilization, pregnancy, recent surgery, thrombophilia, previous DVT etc.
6. Congenital cardiac abnormality.
7. A past history of bleeding disorder, liver disease, previous stroke or diabetes mellitus
8. Smoking and alcohol consumption
9. Family history
10. Findings on examination.
11. Investigations carried out such as a CT /MRI scan, Transcranial Doppler, Trans-oesophageal echo (TOE) or a duplex scan for a DVT and most importantly if a Transcranial Doppler test with agitated saline was carried out to identify a right-to-left shunt

12. The treatment undergone by the patient with subsequent morbidity and mortality.

Identifying the patients and requesting their hospital notes was carried out by the Clinical Effectiveness Unit at Barts and the London NHS Trust and this part of the work took three months.

The prospective study

Based on the above information 15 patients were identified from the original 71 and these were examined in more detail as a prospective study.

All the records were sorted out at the clinical effective unit (clinical governance unit). Medical records were retrieved from the central registry at the Royal London Hospital by myself to get some of the patient's data from the list produced earlier based on the criteria of the study.

The CEU statistician was able to collate the data and present it to us in the form of tables.

Diagnostic Criteria

Those entire patients who were diagnosed with peripheral arterial embolism, thrombosis, and unspecified stroke on the basis of clinical finding and investigation (Duplex scan, TTE, TOE and Agitated saline test) were considered in this study.

Agitated saline test with Transcranial Doppler ultrasound was done on those patients in whom we were suspecting right to left shunt on the basis of information from the questionnaire.

Questionnaire

This was the questionnaire, which was used to obtain data from the 71 patients, as a retrospective study.

Questionnaire About Peripheral Arterial Embolism Due To A Patent Foramen Ovale

General information

NAME
D.O.B
GENDER
RACE
OCCUPATION
D.O.A
D.O.D

Presenting Complaints

Q - 1 What was the main complaint of patient at the time of admission?
if yes please give details:

Arterial embolism in:	Yes	No
Brain (stroke)		
Arm		
Leg		
Bowel		

Q – 2. What was the onset of symptoms.
    Sudden   Gradual

Q – 3. Duration of symptoms.
    Days   Weeks   Months

Q – 4. Was it recurrent?

    Yes   No   N/A

Q – 5. Did the episode occur during :
                           Yes   No   N/A
    Coughing
    Straining at stool
    Sexual intercourse
    Breath holding or
    Any manoeuvre

Q - 6 Was there any predisposing factor for DVT ?
                           Yes   No   N/A
    Immobilization
    Pregnancy
    Recent surgery
    Hypercoagulable state
    Previous DVT
    Others

Past Problems

Q - 7 Was there any congenital cardiac abnormality?
        YES   NO   N/A

Q - 8 Any neurological procedure carried out in childhood?
        YES   NO   N/A

Q - 9 Was there any significant past medical history?
                           YES   NO   N/A
    Bleeding disorder
    Liver disease
    Previous stroke
    Diabetes mellitus
    Others

Q -10 Does the patient smoke?

                    YES   NO   N/A

If yes please
give detail about frequency
of smoking

Q -11 Does the patient drink alcohol?
                    YES   NO   N/A

If yes please
give detail about frequency
of Alcohol drinking

Q -12 Was the same problem running in the family?
        YES   NO   N/A

Q -13 Was there any positive finding on examination?
        YES   NO   N/A

Investigations

Q - 14 Was there any investigation done to screen hypercoagulable state?
        YES   NO   N/A

Q - 15 Was there any investigation done to rule out deep venous thrombosis (DVT)?
        YES   NO   N/A

If yes,
Was it done?

        Within 7 days   Between 8-10 days   After 10 days

Q - 16 what imaging technique was used?
                    YES   NO   N/A
    - CT SCAN
    - MRI
    - Tran cranial

Doppler U/S
　　- Tran's oesophageal
　　　ECHO (TEE)
　　- TEE with agitated saline

Please give detail
If there was any positive information on imaging

Q - 17 What modalities were used to treat the patient?

　　　　　　　YES　　　　　　　NO　　　　　　　N/A

Medical treatment
Surgical treatment
(Embolectomy)

Q - 18 Did the patient survive after treatment?

　　　　　　　YES　　　　　　　NO

Inclusion Criteria

This audit included,
1 - Both male and female patients.
2 - Patients from hospital records.
3 - Patients above 15 years of age.
4 - Known patients with Right to Left shunt due to Patent Foramen Ovale
5 - Admitted or seen as out patients in RLH, LCH, and SBH.
6 - Suspected and confirmed cases of peripheral arterial embolism due to Right to Left Shunt.

Exclusion Criteria

This audit did not include,
1- Patients with the ages less than 15 years.
2- Patients not from the above mentioned hospitals.
3- Patients with known Congenital Heart disease e.g. atrial septal defect (ASD), ventricular septal defect (VSD), tetralogy of Fallot (TOF)
4- Patients with other heart and peripheral vascular disease such as Vasculitis, Raynaud's disease etc

Variables of Interest

- **Demographic trends including occupation:**

Evidence shows that incidence of peripheral arterial (paradoxical) embolism is high in deep-sea divers.

- **Presenting complaints and site of embolism:**

Generally, any organ may be affected by arterial embolism due to a patent foramen ovale but most of patients presented with a stroke of undetermined aetiology.

- **Diagnostic investigations:**

Routine investigations, coagulation profile, Duplex Scan, Angiograms, CT scans, MRI, Trans-thoracic Echocardiography, Trans – oesophageal Echocardiography, Agitated saline test.

- **Management: Surgical or medical**

Embolectomy / anticoagulation

Objectives of the Study

1. To identify arterial embolism patients.

2. Elucidate epidemiology of arterial embolus patients and draw conclusions from this data forming a retrospective study

3. From these patients, identify a sub-group most likely to be suffering from a right to left shunt

4. Review this subgroup of patients in clinic as the prospective part of the study.

5. Arrange Transcranial Agitated saline tests for diagnosis of right-to-left shunt for investigation

Transcranial Doppler Protocol [39]

The Transcranial Doppler and agitated saline test was in the outpatients department at the Royal London hospital with equipment brought from the Homerton Hospital, using the protocol developed at the Homerton and which is reproduced below. This protocol is used in all hospitals in the UK and hence was also used in the clinic organised for the procedure on the selected patients.

Protocol

1. Explain to patient the nature and object of the study. Process involves making an ultrasound recording of blood flow in the brain before and during peripheral venous injection of agitated saline (which contains micro bubbles). Explain that there are no known risks or after effects either from the ultrasound or saline injection and that the procedure will take about 20-30 minutes with no discomfort apart from insertion of a fine cannula (18-20 gauge). Into an arm vein as if for taking a blood sample.

2. Ask questions specified on data form and complete.

3. Prepare patient by making him/her comfortable on a couch and insert a venflon into an arm or hand vein. Connect the venflon to a 3-way stopcock and two 10 ml syringes one of which is filled with normal saline

4. Ask the patient to practice a Valsalva manoeuvre (VM). Patient should be able to forced expire against a closed glottis for 5 seconds. If patient cannot do a VM then use coughing instead.

5. Locate Middle Cerebral Artery using 2 MHz ultrasound probe. Attach headband and relocate MCA. Check that MCA signal stable during VM or coughing.

6. Perform 2-3 recordings. First recording is done at baseline followed by 2 further recordings during VM or coughing. If a micro bubble storm is detected during any of the recordings then the study is positive and complete.

Perform each run as follows;

Time 0-3 seconds inject 10 ml agitated* saline. Start stopwatch:
> Time 5 seconds ask patient to perform a VM/coughing manoeuvre for 5 seconds (only for recordings 2 and 3)
> Time 3-40 run recorder and watch/listen for micro bubbles. If MBs noted run is positive and complete
> Time 120 seconds if no MBs run is negative and complete.

7. Remove venflon and dress cannula site. Offer patient tissue to clean gel from ultrasound site.
8. Print and store report.

*Agitated saline is 10 ml of sterile normal saline pushed back and forth vigorously between the two 10 ml syringes about 10 times. A little air or blood helps micro bubble formation but visible air should not be injected.

The pictures below were all taken with patient knowledge and signed consent:

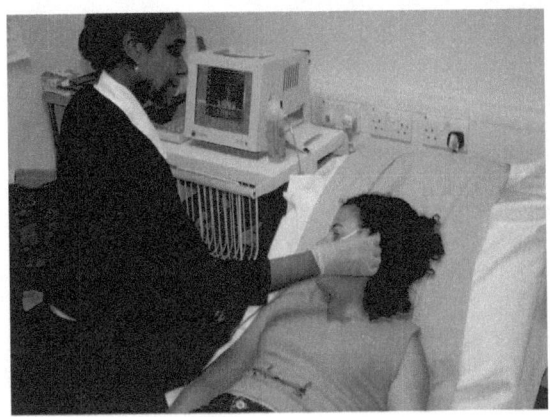

Figure 1 Locating the middle cerebral artery using acoustic coupling medium and an ultrasound probe to locate the artery.

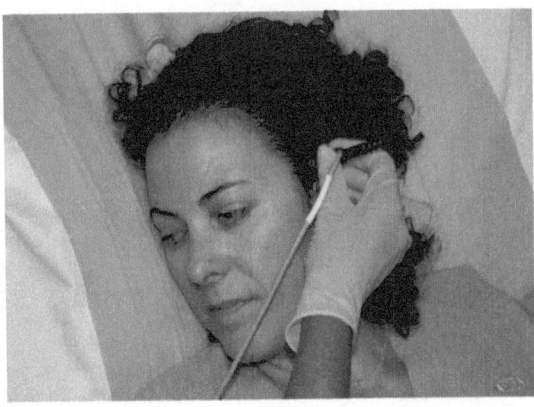

Figure 2 Locating the middle cerebral artery and making sure the signals stay stable during VM or coughing.

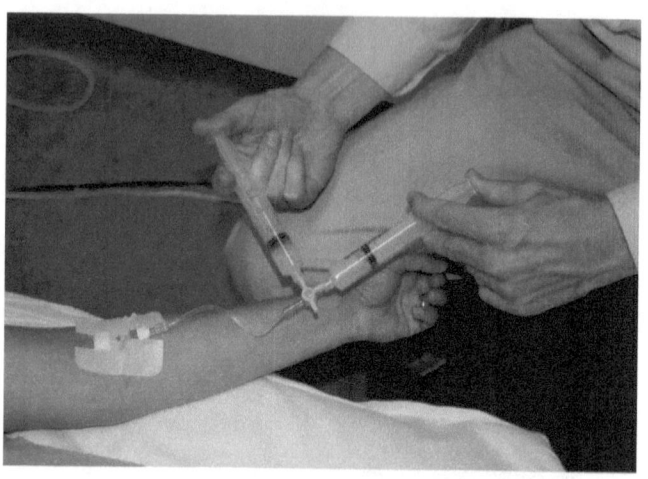

Figure 3 Agitated saline pushed back and forth vigorously between the two 10ml syringes about 10 times. Visible air should not be injected.

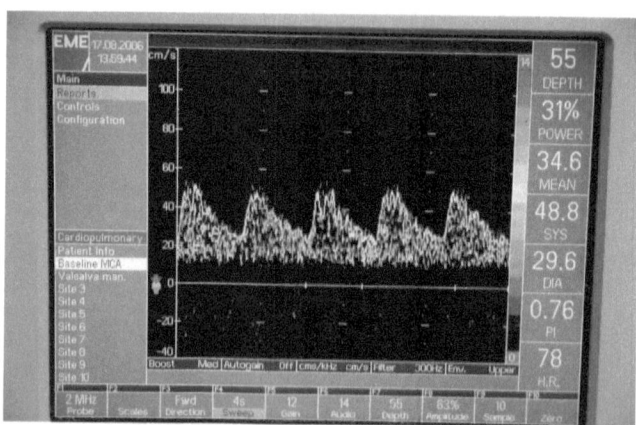

Figure 4 Transcranial Doppler shunt study recording the middle cerebral artery flow through the skull before intravenous microbubbles injection.

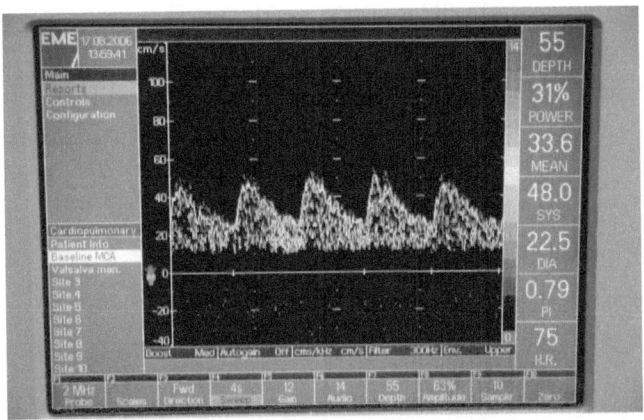

Figure 5 Transcranial Doppler readings of middle cerebral artery during the valsalva manoeuvre. Reading kept stable for the procedure to proceed.

The patient shown in the photographs was not a part of the present study but she was found to have a paradoxical embolism due to a PFO.

On the basis of the prospective study only five from the 15 patients were available for the procedure, 3 from the 15 had already had a percutaneous closure of PFO and unfortunately seven were not available.

The results from the procedure were written into a format as shown below.

SURNAME   FORENAME
DATE OF BIRTH   GENDER
HOSPITAL   CONSULTANT
NUMBER

Transcranial Doppler for Right to Left Cardiopulmonary Shunt

DATE OF STUDY

INDICATION

FINDINGS

Baseline response to agitated saline   0

Valsalva 1 response to agitated saline   0

Valsalva 2 response to agitated saline   0

0 = no microbubbles   1 = 1 - 20   2 = >20 no shower   3 = >20 with shower

CONCLUSION

Results

Retrospective study

Results obtained from the notes on the 71 patients were processed statistically.

The results were grouped into form of tables, which are as follows:

Table 1 Gender

Gender

		Frequency	Percent
Valid	Male	44	62.0
	Female	27	38.0
	Total	71	100.0

44 were males and 27 out of the 71 patients were females.

Table 2 Age

Statistics

age1

N	Valid	70
	Missing	1
Mean		65.10
Minimum		2
Maximum		96

The age range was 2- 96, with the mean age being 65.1yrs

Table 3 Occupation

Occupation

		Frequency	Percent
Valid	Chef	1	1.4
	Child!	1	1.4
	Ex-Royal Artillery man	1	1.4
	Long distance lorry driver	1	1.4
	N/D	53	74.6
	P/T work	1	1.4
	Previous ticket office worker	1	1.4
	Retired	10	14.1
	Scuber diver - now jobless	1	1.4
	Unemployed	1	1.4
	Total	71	100.0

No conclusions regarding the importance of occupation on the prevalence of an arterial embolus could be made from this data since so many patients' occupations were unrecorded in the notes. Only one was a scuba diver, which holds relevance for this study, as a PFO if present would allow air bubbles to pass into the arterial circulation, which would create complications.

Table 4 Location of arterial embolism / pain

Location of arterial embolism/pain

		Frequency	Percent
Valid	Brain (stroke)	1	1.4
	Arm	5	7.0
	Leg	36	50.7
	Foot/heel	9	12.7
	Leg + foot	3	4.2
	Plapitations/chest pain/SOB	2	2.8
	Hip/leg/abdo	1	1.4
	Peripheral vascular disease + transient cerebral ischemia	1	1.4
	Peripheral vascular disease/Intermittent claudication	1	1.4
	Intermittent claudication/occluded eight superficial femoral artery	1	1.4
	Peripheral vascular disease/hypertension	1	1.4
	Buttocks	1	1.4
	Access related problem	1	1.4
	Recurrent cough, hoarseness of voice, AAA	1	1.4
	Respiratory infection	1	1.4
	Clotted fistula	1	1.4
	Intermittent claudication	1	1.4
	Difficulty walking	1	1.4
	Peripheral vascular disease	1	1.4
	Leg + arm	2	2.8
	Total	71	100.0

The frequency was highest for the presence of an embolism in the leg (36 patients, just over half the sample). The lower limbs showed a higher incidence of an arterial embolism when compared to the rest. The reason for this is probably that half the cardiac output goes to the legs.

Table 5 Onset of symptoms

What was the onset of symptoms

		Frequency	Percent
Valid	Sudden	21	29.6
	Gradual	50	70.4
	Total	71	100.0

70.4 % of the patients had a gradual onset when compared to 29.6 % of patients who had a sudden onset of symptoms.

Table 6 Duration of complaints

How long has the patient been having these complaints

		Frequency	Percent
Valid	Days	13	18.3
	Weeks	14	19.7
	Months	41	57.7
	N/D	2	2.8
	Years	1	1.4
	Total	71	100.0

The duration of symptoms varied; days were found in 13 patients had been suffering for less than a week, 14 for between a week and a month, and 41 for more than a month. 2 patients were not documented.

Table 7 Frequency of symptoms

Was it recurrent

		Frequency	Percent
Valid	Yes	45	63.4
	No	24	33.8
	N/A	2	2.8
	Total	71	100.0

A higher percentage of the patients had a recurrence of signs and symptoms and around 34 percent had no recurrence after treatment given.

Table 8 Cause of embolus

Complaint happened due to

		Frequency	Percent
Valid	Coughing	1	1.4
	Exercise/walking	7	9.9
	Not asked/Not documented	32	45.1
	None / N/A	29	40.8
	Elevation	1	1.4
	Stopped Warfarin 3/52 ago	1	1.4
	Total	71	100.0

Unfortunately about 85% of the records did not contain information on the cause of the embolus; the remaining 15% were associated with coughing, exercise/walking, elevation of leg and cessation of anticoagulation.

Table 9 Immobilisation

Any predisposing factor of DVT - immobilization

		Frequency	Percent
Valid	Yes	12	16.9
	No	52	73.2
	Not asked or N/D	4	5.6
	N/A	3	4.2
	Total	71	100.0

12 were immobilized which lead to a DVT.

Table 10 Pregnancy

Any predisposing factor of DVT - pregnancy

		Frequency	Percent
Valid	No	63	88.7
	Not asked or N/D	5	7.0
	N/A	3	4.2
	Total	71	100.0

None of the females from the 71 patients were found to be pregnant.

Table 11 Recent Surgery

Any predisposing factor of DVT - recent surgery

		Frequency	Percent
Valid	Yes	16	22.5
	No	47	66.2
	Not asked or N/D	6	8.5
	N/A	2	2.8
	Total	71	100.0

Recent surgery does play an important part in the formation of a DVT and we found that 16 patients were affected from the same.

Table 12 Hypercoaguble state

Any predisposing factor of DVT - hypercoaguble state

		Frequency	Percent
Valid	Yes	14	19.7
	No	50	70.4
	Not asked or N/D	5	7.0
	N/A	2	2.8
	Total	71	100.0

Around 20% had hypercoaguability as a predisposing factor of DVT.

Table 13 Previous DVT

Any predisposing factor of DVT - previous DVT

		Frequency	Percent
Valid	Yes	10	14.1
	No	53	74.6
	Not asked or N/D	6	8.5
	N/A	2	2.8
	Total	71	100.0

DVT as we know has a high recurrence rate and in the present study ten patients had a recurrence.

Table 14 Other Predisposing factors of a DVT

Any predisposing factor of DVT - others

		Frequency	Percent
Valid	Yes	20	28.2
	No	43	60.6
	Not asked or N/D	6	8.5
	N/A	2	2.8
	Total	71	100.0

While in the others group we found 20 patients to be affected.

Summarizing the causes and the statistical analysis of the predisposing factors of DVT; the predisposing factors taken into consideration were immobilization, pregnancy, recent surgery, hypercoagulable state, previous DVT, others.

None of the patients were pregnant – not a surprising finding considering the high average age and the preponderance of males in the sample; a higher frequency was seen for patients who had undergone recent surgery and with other predisposing factors. Around 20 percent had hypercoagubility as a factor and around fourteen percent of the patients had either a previous DVT, or were immobilized.

Summing up, 53 patients (75%) had a predisposing factor leading to DVT.

Table 15 Congenital abnormalities

Any congenital abnormality since childhood

		Frequency	Percent
Valid	No	11	15.5
	Not asked	28	39.4
	Not noted	19	26.8
	N/A	13	18.3
	Total	71	100.0

Statistically from the table above the actual number patients who did not have any congenital abnormality were eleven whilst the rest had no documented data for analysis.

Table 16 Neurological procedures

Any neurological procedure carried out in childhood

		Frequency	Percent
Valid	Yes	2	2.8
	No	13	18.3
	Not asked	28	39.4
	Not noted	16	22.5
	N/A	12	16.9
	Total	71	100.0

There was no patient in the group with a congenital abnormality and only 2 patients had procedure carried out in childhood, though the majority had no data on paper.

Table 17 Bleeding disorders

Any significant past medical history - bleeding disorder

		Frequency	Percent
Valid	Yes	2	2.8
	No	64	90.1
	Not asked/not documented	4	5.6
	N/A	1	1.4
	Total	71	100.0

Only two patients in this group had a bleeding disorder.

Table 18 Liver disease

Any significant past medical history - liver disease

		Frequency	Percent
Valid	Yes	2	2.8
	No	64	90.1
	Not asked/not documented	4	5.6
	N/A	1	1.4
	Total	71	100.0

Although 40% of the 71 patients consumed alcohol, only two suffered from liver disease.

Table 19 Previous stroke

Any significant past medical history - previous stroke

		Frequency	Percent
Valid	Yes	5	7.0
	No	61	85.9
	Not asked/not documented	4	5.6
	N/A	1	1.4
	Total	71	100.0

As mentioned earlier about the risk of a transient ischaemic attack or stroke in association with a PFO, we found five to have suffered from a previous attack and out these five patients one was suspected to have a PFO. This patient's agitated saline test was negative.

Table 20 Diabetes Mellitus

Any significant past medical history - diabetes mellitus

		Frequency	Percent
Valid	Yes	15	21.1
	No	52	73.2
	Not asked/not documented	3	4.2
	N/A	1	1.4
	Total	71	100.0

This reflects the high proportion of these patients who suffer from diabetes.

Table 21 Other past medical histories

Any significant past medical history - others

		Frequency	Percent
Valid	Yes	52	73.2
	No	17	23.9
	Not asked/not documented	1	1.4
	N/A	1	1.4
	Total	71	100.0

73% of the patients had a significant past medical history.

As far as a significant past medical history is concerned; about 21 percent of the patients had a history of Diabetes mellitus and seven percent had a stroke. Bleeding and liver disorders were a minimum being less than 5%. Most patients fell in the 'others' group of past medical history.

Table 22 Smoking

History of smoking

		Frequency	Percent
Valid	Yes	48	67.6
	No	17	23.9
	Not asked	1	1.4
	N/D	5	7.0
	Total	71	100.0

Nicotine predisposes to DVT. 67.6% of the selected patients were smokers.

Table 23 Frequency of smoking

If yes, how many

		Frequency	Percent
Valid	>20/day	1	1.4
	1/day	1	1.4
	10-20/day 53 yrs	1	1.4
	10/day for 20 yrs	1	1.4
	15/day for 35 yrs	1	1.4
	2 ounces/month	1	1.4
	20-30/day for 20 yrs	1	1.4
	20/day	8	11.3
	3/day for 10yrs	1	1.4
	3/day since surgery	1	1.4
	30 yrs 30-40/day	1	1.4
	40/day	1	1.4
	40/day yrs	1	1.4
	5/day	2	2.8
	56g tobacco/weed for past 10 yrs	1	1.4
	Ex - 1993	1	1.4
	ex - 20/day stopped 20 yrs ago	1	1.4
	Ex	3	4.2
	Ex >20 yrs	1	1.4
	Ex 25 yrs ago	1	1.4
	Ex 8/day	1	1.4
	Ex smoker	3	4.2
	Ex smoker 20/day for 30 yrs	1	1.4
	Ex smoker 40/d	1	1.4
	N/A	17	23.9
	N/D	2	2.8
	Not noted	14	19.7
	Pack/day 20 yrs	1	1.4
	Roll ups	1	1.4
	Total	71	100.0

From the detailed history of the amount of smoking carried out, the prominent number, which came into picture, was for smokers smoking 20 cigarettes per day, which were eight. Two of the smokers from the 71 patients smoked five cigarettes per day, whilst 9 were ex-smokers and the remainder had varying frequencies of the amount of nicotine they smoked as mentioned in the table above.

Table 24 Alcohol consumption

History of alcohol drinking

		Frequency	Percent
Valid	Yes	27	38.0
	No	34	47.9
	Not asked	3	4.2
	Not noted	7	9.9
	Total	71	100.0

Alcohol has a varying effect on the vascular tree depending on the dose. It was found that 27 consumed alcohol.

Table 25 Frequency of Alcohol consumption

If yes, details

		Frequency	Percent
Valid	10 pints/wk	1	1.4
	2/3 cans larger/day	1	1.4
	4-5 litres/day	1	1.4
	5/6 cans of larger/day	1	1.4
	Alcoholic drinker	1	1.4
	Binge	1	1.4
	Ez drinker	1	1.4
	N/A	41	57.7
	N/D	1	1.4
	Not noted	7	9.9
	Occassionaly	12	16.9
	Rarely	1	1.4
	Usually heavy drinking	1	1.4
	Wk + evening	1	1.4
	Total	71	100.0

From the 27 who consumed alcohol 12 drank occasionally, though only a few were heavy drinkers.

Percentages wise to summarize 67.6 % were smokers and around 38% drank alcohol.

Table 26 Family history

Does the same problem run in the family

		Frequency	Percent
Valid	Yes	9	12.7
	No	25	35.2
	Not asked	15	21.1
	Not noted	12	16.9
	N/A	10	14.1
	Total	71	100.0

Only 9 patients had a positive family history.

Table 27 Positive signs

Any positive finding on examination

		Frequency	Percent
Valid	Yes	60	84.5
	No	3	4.2
	Not documented	6	8.5
	N/A	2	2.8
	Total	71	100.0

84.5 % showed a positive fining on examination.

Table 28 Hypercoagulable state screening

Any investigation done to screen hypercoagulable state

		Frequency	Percent
Valid	Yes	41	57.7
	No	23	32.4
	Not asked	1	1.4
	N/D	5	7.0
	N/A	1	1.4
	Total	71	100.0

57.7% of the patients underwent an investigation for a hypercoagulable state where as 32.4 % of patients did not.

Table 29 Ruling out DVT

Any investigation done to rule out DVT

		Frequency	Percent
Valid	Yes	32	45.1
	No	28	39.4
	Not asked	1	1.4
	Not noted	7	9.9
	N/A	3	4.2
	Total	71	100.0

There were 32 patients who underwent an investigation to rule out DVT

Table 30 Time duration of DVT screening

If yes, when was this carried out

		Frequency	Percent
Valid	Within 7 days	17	23.9
	Between 8-10 days	3	4.2
	After 10 days	5	7.0
	N/A	31	43.7
	Not noted	15	21.1
	Total	71	100.0

32 patients who had an investigation done to rule out DVT and it was important to know when the test was carried out. 23.9% of them had it done within 7 days that plays an important part of the study. Two patients had it between 8-10 days and 5 after 10 days.

Table 31 Imagining techniques

What imaging technique was carried out

		Frequency	Percent
Valid	Tran cranial doppler U/S	5	7.0
	Tran's oesophageal ECHO (TEE)	6	8.5
	N/D / none	9	12.7
	Other	3	4.2
	Tran cranial doppler U/S + other	2	2.8
	MRI, TEE, TEE with agitated saline	1	1.4
	Duplex	4	5.6
	Angiogram/Angioplasty	12	16.9
	Echocardiogram	4	5.6
	ECG	2	2.8
	Arterial duplex scan + angiogram	2	2.8
	Multiple	2	2.8
	Doppler + Tran's oesophageal	1	1.4
	MRI + TEE	1	1.4
	ECHO + angioplasty	2	2.8
	B/L veinogram	1	1.4
	ECG, Angio, Duplex	1	1.4
	CT, MRI + TEE	1	1.4
	Multiple!	2	2.8
	Doppler, TEE + TEE with saline	1	1.4
	Angiogram + CT	1	1.4
	CT, Duplex and ECHO	1	1.4
	Ultrasound + doppler	1	1.4
	Doppler + angiogram	1	1.4
	TEE + Duplex	1	1.4
	Duplex, Angiogram, CT scan + TEE	1	1.4
	Angiogram, TEE + ECHO	1	1.4
	None	1	1.4
	Duplex, TTE + TOE	1	1.4
	Total	71	100.0

The majority underwent an angiogram or an angioplasty. Transcranial Doppler, duplex and echocardiogram all had the same individual percentage of frequency of the test carried out 9 % of the patients had a TOE done.

Around 4 % individually had either a Transcranial Doppler, ECG, Arterial duplex scan or angiogram. While MRI, TEE, TEE with agitated saline, Doppler + Transoesophageal, MRI +TEE, ECHO + angioplasty, B/L veinogram, ECG, Angiogram, Duplex, CT, MRI + TEE, Doppler, TEE + TEE with saline and Angiogram + CT.

Table 32 Treatment modalities

What modalities were used to treat the patient

		Frequency	Percent
Valid	Medical treatment	21	29.6
	Surgical treatment	35	49.3
	No treatment documented	3	4.2
	Both	12	16.9
	Total	71	100.0

Table 33 Mortality

Did the patient survive after treatment

		Frequency	Percent
Valid	Yes	60	84.5
	No	1	1.4
	N/D	10	14.1
	Total	71	100.0

Treatment wise, 50% had surgical treatment, 30% medical and 17% had both modalities. Only one death was reported after the treatment given.

Prospective study results

From the 71 patients included in the study having a peripheral arterial embolus, 15 of these were selected or were presumed to have a right to left shunt and they were then brought into a special clinic organised to test if they had the same. The result for the agitated saline test, which was carried out on five of these patients, is mentioned below:

Table 34 Agitated saline testing

Agitated Saline Test done

		Frequency	Percent
	Yes - result negative	15	21.1
Valid	No	56	78.9
	Total	71	100.0

The agitated saline tests using the transcranial Doppler were carried out at the Royal London Hospital on two occasions.

Of the 12 patients, only five were available for the test.

Consent was taken and procedure explained, full aseptic measures were taken and the test performed.

All five tests were negative and no right-to-left shunts were found.

The format of the report

SURNAME **FORENAME**
DATE OF BIRTH **GENDER**
HOSPITAL NUMBER **CONSULTANT**

TRANSCRANIAL DOPPLER FOR RIGHT TO LEFT CARDIOPULMONARY SHUNT

DATE OF STUDY

INDICATION

FINDINGS MIDDLE CEREBRAL ARTERY IMAGING
Baseline response to agitated saline — 0
Valsalva 1 response to agitated saline — 0
Valsalva 2 response to agitated saline — 0
0 = no microbubbles   1 = 1-20   2 = >20 no shower   3 = >20 with shower

CONCLUSION

The following are the reports of the 5 patients who under went the procedure:

Report for patient number 1

SURNAME	1.	**FORENAME**	
DATE OF BIRTH	25/05/1951	**GENDER**	Female
HOSPITAL NUMBER		**CONSULTANT**	

Transcranial Doppler for Right to Left Cardiopulmonary Shunt

DATE OF STUDY 14th June 2006

INDICATION Suspected Patent foramen ovale

FINDINGS MIDDLE CEREBRAL ARTERY IMAGING
Baseline response to 0 agitated saline
Valsalva 1 response to 0 agitated saline
Valsalva 2 response to 0 agitated saline
0 = no microbubbles   1 = 1 - 20   2 = >20 no shower   3 = >20 with shower

CONCLUSION NEGATIVE FOR RIGHT TO LEFT CARDIOPULMONARY SHUNT.

Report for patient number 2

SURNAME	2.	**FORENAME**	
DATE OF BIRTH	25/05/1951	**GENDER**	Male
HOSPITAL NUMBER		**CONSULTANT**	

Transcranial Doppler for Right to Left Cardiopulmonary Shunt

DATE OF STUDY 28th June 2006

INDICATION Suspected right to left shunt.

FINDINGS MIDDLE CEREBRAL ARTERY IMAGING
Baseline response to agitated saline 0
Valsalva 1 response to agitated saline 0
Valsalva 2 response to agitated saline 0

0 = no microbubbles 1 = 1 - 20 2 = >20 no shower 3 = >20 with shower

CONCLUSION NEGATIVE FOR RIGHT TO LEFT CARDIOPULMONARY SHUNT.

Report for patient number 3

SURNAME	3.	**FORENAME**	
DATE OF BIRTH	03/12/1961	**GENDER**	Female
HOSPITAL NUMBER		**CONSULTANT**	

Transcranial Doppler for Right to Left Cardiopulmonary Shunt

DATE OF STUDY   14th June 2006

INDICATION   Postpartum CVA, Previous left brachial embolectomy

FINDINGS   MIDDLE CEREBRAL ARTERY IMAGING
Baseline response to 0 agitated saline
Valsalva 1 response to 0 agitated saline
Valsalva 2 response to 0 agitated saline

0 = no microbubbles   1 = 1 - 20   2 = >20 no shower   3 = >20 with shower

CONCLUSION   NEGATIVE FOR RIGHT TO LEFT CARDIOPULMONARY SHUNT.

Report for patient number 4

SURNAME	4.	**FORENAME**	
DATE OF BIRTH	14/05/1944	**GENDER**	Male
HOSPITAL NUMBER	(Royal London)	**CONSULTANT**	

Transcranial Doppler for Right to Left Cardiopulmonary Shunt

DATE OF STUDY   14th June 2006

INDICATION   DVT

FINDINGS   MIDDLE CEREBRAL ARTERY IMAGING
Baseline response to agitated saline — 0
Valsalva 1 response to agitated saline — 0
Valsalva 2 response to agitated saline — 0
0 = no microbubbles   1 = 1 - 20   2 = >20 no shower   3 = >20 with shower

CONCLUSION   NEGATIVE FOR RIGHT TO LEFT CARDIOPULMONARY SHUNT.

Report for patient number 5

SURNAME	5.	**FORENAME**	
DATE OF BIRTH	25/04/1940	**GENDER**	Female
HOSPITAL NUMBER		**CONSULTANT**	Mr.Cross

Transcranial Doppler for Right to Left Cardiopulmonary Shunt

DATE OF STUDY 14th June 2006

INDICATION Bachet's syndrome

FINDINGS MIDDLE CEREBRAL ARTERY IMAGING
Baseline response to 0 agitated saline
Valsalva 1 response to 0 agitated saline
Valsalva 2 response to 0 agitated saline
0 = no microbubbles   1 = 1 - 20   2 = >20 no shower   3 = >20 with shower

CONCLUSION NEGATIVE FOR RIGHT TO LEFT CARDIOPULMONARY SHUNT.

None of the patients tested had a right to left shunt. It was presumed that though attaining the percentage of 25-30% in the general population who have a PFO we could have missed out on patients who actually had one on the basis of the small number of this study. Hence a bigger prospective study would be beneficial later on to come to a more reliable result.

The retrospective study mirrors the risk factors for vascular disease and the findings are compatible with similar larger studies in the literature 73,74.

Discussion

The present study showed that PFO may not be a major or direct cause of paradoxical embolism, even though there is direct evidence dating back to 1877 that this might be the case.[40, 41]

Many studies show that there is a high prevalence of PFO present in approximately one-quarter of the general population.[42, 43] Age does not play much of a role on the formation of an embolus and is not a predictor of PFO in patients with cerebral ischaemic events.[5] In the present study the mean age was 65.1 years and none of them were found to have a PFO (RLS). The three patients who we reviewed who had already had PFO closures were all below 55 years of age. Also there have been studies showing that ASA and PFO are frequently observed with cerebral ischaemic events especially in patients who are less than 55 years old[44, 45].

Paradoxical embolism through a PFO is a recognised cause of stroke (cryptogenic/transient)[46, 47]. In our small study, very few patients had suffered a properly diagnosed stroke. In a recent study in Minnesota U.S.A[48] which concluded that "Patent foramen ovale is not a risk factor for cryptogenic ischaemic stroke or transient ischaemic attack in the general population."

There was one occupational scuba diver included in our study, though he did not show any signs of PFO. There are studies which show that PFO increases the risk for decompression illness by a factor of up to 5 times due to the increase in intrathoracic pressure.[49, 50, 51]. These subjects should minimise the load of tissue nitrogen during dives or if this is not possible they should give up diving[51].

An embolus can be found anywhere in the circulatory tree but half the patients in the present study had a leg embolus.
A high percentage (63.4%) of patients had recurrence of symptoms, which suggests that regular checkups are necessary and definite treatment, either medical or surgical, is necessary.

Many had predisposing factors for DVT, such as immunization, a hypercoagulable state or recent surgery. It is presumed that the mechanism for PFO-related systemic ischaemic events is paradoxical embolization of thromboembolic fragments originating from the venous tree [40]. Hence paradoxical embolism could be a risk of DVT.

Deep venous thrombosis was detected in nearly 10% of patients with PFO as the sole identifiable cardiac risk factor and it was suggested that phlebography should be performed in patients with medium or large interatrial shunts if a paradoxical embolism is suspected[52]. It was also recorded in a study that approximately 30% of stroke patients subsequently develop a DVT secondary to stroke[53] but the mechanism in these cases is presumably related to stasis following paralysis.

It was found in the present study that 67.6% of our patients were smokers and around 40% of the patients were alcoholics.

Smoking, diabetes mellitus and a positive family history are all moderate risk factors for venous thromboembolism[54]. A positive finding of the signs of postphlebitic limb is often found on examination and here 84.5% of our patients exhibited this. Investigations for thrombophilia should be carried out and in our retrospective study of 71 patients we found that only half of the patients had undergone this investigation.

There has been much debate on the ideal investigation to rule out a PFO or other right-to-left shunt. Contrast trans-oesophageal echo, a semi-invasive technique, has been regarded as the gold standard for the detection of PFO[55, 56, 57].

In this study 9% of the patients underwent TOE. MRI, TTE and TOE with agitated saline test were performed on only one patient. Doppler + TOE were also carried out on one patient.

Doppler, TTE + TOE with agitated saline contrast were performed on just one patient. Recent studies show that c-TTE with second harmonic imaging and c-TOE are equivalent in sensitivity.[57, 58, 59]. The same study showed that c-TOE was not perfect for the diagnosis as sedation is used, hindering the valsalva manoeuver [18]; which is a safe and useful technique to detect the presence of PFO [60].

Contrast transcranial doppler (c-TCD) has found to be very sensitive in the detection of a RLS [57, 61], and when compared to c-TOE its sensitivity appears to be high[57, 62, 63]. In the present study we found around 7% who had a TCD done and 12 patients were selected on whom TCD with saline was carried out. One study showed that it was as sensitive as c-TOE.[64, 65]

This means that there is a significant possibility of false positive results showing up with the TCD technique[18]. Trancranial Doppler augmented by power M-mode ultrasound is a new technology allowing improved display features and enhancing sensitivity to contrast bubble emboli over single-gated TCD examination.[65, 66, 67]

Of the 71 patients in the retrospective study a quarter was treated medically and half were treated surgically while 16.9% had both forms of treatment. One patient died before the treatment was started.

Percutaneous closure of PFO with atrial septal aneurysm (ASA) is a minimally invasive procedure, safe, effective in the prevention of recurrent strokes, avoiding life long anticoagulants and also cures migraine to some extent.[68, 69]

Conclusions

Apparently there is an incidence of PFO (Right to left shunt) in patients with peripheral arterial embolism, but our study shows that it could not be a major cause of undiagnosed peripheral arterial embolism.

Our results conform to the accepted incidence of PFO at an estimated percentage of 25-30% [70, 71, 72] in the general population.

Male smokers probably have a higher incidence of paradoxical embolism in the lower limbs with predisposing factors leading to a DVT.

Future Proposals

The conclusion of the study was a negative result; PFO may not be a major cause of undiagnosed paradoxical arterial embolism; the incidence of PFO in our patients was the same as in the general population.

Any future study would be a small prospective study, which would investigate all arterial embolus patients attending an A & E department for right-to-left shunt. In order for this to be a meaningful study several hospitals would need to be recruited.

References

1. S.G. Fransson. The Botallo Mystery, Clin Cardiol 22(1999):434- 436.
2. Sandy Shah, Daniel Shindler, Facc et al, Patent Foramen Ovale- Current concepts, New Jersey Medicine, June 2002, 99(6):25-26
3. Tushar Chatterjee, Michael Petzsch, Huseyin Ince et al, Interventional Closure with Amplatzer PFO occluder of patent foramen ovale in patient with Paradoxical cereberal embolism; Journal of interventional Radiology, Vol 18, No. 3. 2005: 137-179.
4. Asif Hasan, Anjum, parvez, Mr Ajmal et al Clinical significance JIACM Dec 2004, 5(4):339-44
5. P.H. Lechat et al. 'Prevalence of Patent Foramen Ovale in patient with stroke," N Engl. J Med 318(1988):1148-1152.
6. M. W. Webster et al 'patent Foramen Ovale in Young Stroke Patients," Lancet 2(1988): 11-12
7. D. Ranoux et al. 'Patent Foramen Ovale: Is Stroke Due to Paradoxical Embolism?" Stroke 24(1993):31-34
8. J.L. Mas and M. Zuber. " Recurrent Cerebrovascular Events in patient with patent foramen ovale, Arterial septal aneurysm, or both and cryptogenic Stroke or Transient Ischemic Attack. Am Heart J130(1995):1083-1088.
9. J. Bogousslavsky et al. "Stroke Recurrence in patients with patent foramen ovale: The Lusanne Study," Neurology 46(1996):1301-1305.
10. B. Cujec, R. Mainra, and D.H.Johnson. " Prevention of Recurrent cereberal ischemic events in patients with patent foramen ovale and cryptogenic Strokes or Transient Ischemic Attacks. Can J Cardiol 15, no.1 (1999):57-64.
11. D. Stone et al. Patent Foramen Ovale: Association between the degree of shunt by contrast Transesophageal Echocardiography and the Risk of future Ischemic Neurologic events. Am Heart J 131 (1996)158-161
12. Lynch JJ, Schuchard GH, Gross CM, Wann LS. Prevalence of Right to left atrial shunting in a healthy population: detection by Valsalva manoeuvre contrast echocardiography. Am J Cardiol. 1984; 53: 1478-1480.

13. Meissner I, Whisnant JP, Khandhena BK, et al. Prevalence of potential risk factors for stroke assessed by trans-esophageal echocardiography and carotid ultrasonography: the SPARC study: (Stroke prevention: Assessment of risk in a community). Mayo clin Proc. 1999; 74:862-869

14. Lethen H, Flachskampf FA, Schneider R, et al, Frequency of deep venous thrombosis in patients with patent foramen ovale and ischemic attack. Am J Cardiol. (1997): 1066-1069.

15. Vuyisile T N Komo, Pierre Theume calin V Maniu, Krishna Swamy Chandra Sekaran, et al, Patent Foaramen Ovale Tran catheter closure device thrombosis. Rochester. Oct 2001 Vol. 76, iss 10: 1057-1062

16. P. Siostrzonek et al. "Comparison of Transesophageal and Transthoracic Contrast Echocardiography for Detection of a Patent Foramen Ovale," Am J Cardiol 68 (991):1247-1249

17. D. Hausmann, A. Mugge, and W. G. Daniel. " I dentification of patent foramen ovale permitting paradoxical embolism,"J Am Coll Cardiol 26(1995):1030-1038

18. M. Guffi et al. "Surgical Prophylaxis of recurrent stroke in patient with patent foramen ovale: A Pilot study. J Thoracic Cardiovasc Surg 112(1996): 260-263.

19. G. Devuyst et al. " Prognosis after Stroke followed by Surgical Closure of Patent Foramen Ovale: A prospective follow up study with brain MRI and simultaneous Trans-esophageal and Trans- cranial Doppler Ultrasound. Neurology 47(1996): 1162-1166

20. P. Ruchat et al. " Systemic surgical closure of patent foramen ovale in selected patient with Cerebrovascular Events Due to Paradoxical Embolism: Early Results of Preliminary Study, " E J Cardio- thoracic Surgery11(1997):824-827

21. N. Bridges et al. "Tran- catheter Closure of patent foramen ovale after presumed Paradoxical embolism," Circulation 86(1992):1902-1908.

22. H. Sievert et al. " Trans-catheter Closure of Atrial Septal Defect and patent foramen ovale with the Asdos Device(A multi- institutional European Trial)," Am J Cardiol 82(1998): 1495-1413.

23. S. Windecker et al. "Percutaneous Closure of patent foramen ovale in patients with paradoxical embolism Long term risk of Recurrent Thromboembolic events. Circulation 101(2000): 893-898.

24. Meir B, Lock JE, et al. Contemporary management of Patent Foramen Ovale. Circulatin.2003; (107): 5-9.
25. Meissner I, Whishnant J, Khandheria BK, et al. Prevalence of potential risk factors for stroke assessed by transoesophageal echocardiography and carotid ultra sonography: The SPARC Study, Mayo Clinic Proc 1999; 74 :862-869
26. Holmes Dr Jr, Cabalka A. Was your mother Right do, we always need to close the door? Circulation 2002; 106: 1034-1036
27. Harold P AdamsJr, patent foramen ovale : Paradoxical Embolism and Paradoxical data. R ochester: Jan 2004. 79(1), pg 15
28. Lamy C, giannesini C, Zuber M et al. Clinical and imaging finding in cryptogenic stroke patient with or ith out patent foramen ovale; The PFO-ASA study – Atrial Septal Aneurysm stroke. 2003; (33): 706-711.
29. Oliver K, Mohrs Steffen E, Petersen Damir, Erkapic et al: Diagnosis of patent framen ovale using contrast enhancd dynamic MRI(pilot study): AJR: 184 Jan 2005
30. Kessel-Schaefer A, Lefkovits M, Zellweger MJ, et al. Migrating thrombus trapped in a patent foramen ovale. Circulation 2001; 103:1928
31. Manolo Beelke,Silvia Angeli, Massimo Del Sette,Carlo Gandolfo,et al. Prevelnce of patent foramen ovale in subjects with obstructive sleep apnea: a trancranial doppler ultrasound study.
32. Beelke M, Angeli S, Del Sette M,et al.Obstructive sleep apnea can be provocative for right to left shunting through a PFO. Sleep 2002;25:856-62
33. Lavie P.Incidence of sleep apnea in a presumably healthy working population:a significant relationship with excessive day time sleepiness. Sleep 1983;6:312-8
34. Young TJ,Palta M, Dempsey J, et al.The occurrence of sleep-disordered breathing among middle aged adults.N Engl J Med 1993;382:1230-5
35. N.Morelli,S Gori,G.Cafforio.et al. Prevelence of right –to-left shunt in patients with cluster headache.
36. Del.Sette M,Angeli S, Leandri M, et al. Migraine with aura and right to left shunt on trancranial doppler: a case control study.1998.

37. Sztajzel R, Genoud D, Roth S, et al. Le Floch-Rohr J (2002) Patent foramen ovale, a possible cause of symptomatic migraine: a study of 74 patients with acute ischemic stroke. Cerebrovasc Dis 13:102-106
38. Angeli S, Del Sette M, Beelke M, et al. Trancranial doppler in the diagnosis of cardiac patent foramen ovale. 2001.Neurol Sci 22: 353-356.
39. Hommerton hospital, department of cardiovascular surgery. W.Arshad, Kurban.
40. T.Chatterjee M.D.,M. Petzsch,M.D., H. Ince, M.D et al.Interventional Closure with PFO occluder of patent foramen ovale in patients with Paradoxical cerebral embolism. (J Interven Cardiol 2005;18:173-179)
41. Cohnheim J. Thrombose und Embolie. Vorlesung uber Allgemeine Pathologie. Bd 1. Berlin Hirschwald, 1877,175-176.
42. Hagen PT, Scholz DG, Edwards WD. Incidence and size of patetn foramen ovale during the first 10 decades of life: An autopsy study of 965 normal hearts.Mayo clinic proc 1984;59:17-20.
43. E. Ontorato,M.D., G.Melzi,M.D., F. Casilli,M.D., et al. patent foramen ovale with paradoxical embolism : Mid-term resuls of Transcatheter closure in 256 patients. (J Interven cardiol 2003;16:43-50)
44. Abutaher M.YAhia,M.D., A.Shaukat,M.D.,M.P.h., Jawad F. Kirmani,M.D et al. Age is not a predictor of Patent foramen ovale with right-to-left shunt in patients with cerebral ischemic events.(Echocardiography, Volume 21, August 2004).
45. Cujec B, Mainra R, Johnson DH: Prevention of recurrent cerebral ischemic events in patients with patent foramen ovale and cryptogenic strokes or transient ischemic attacks. Can J Cardiol 1999; 15:57-64.
46. Nagno K, Otsubo R, Yasaka M,et al. Stroke recurrence in patients with brain embolism and patent foramen ovale—association with deep vein thrombosis detected by ultrasonography. Rinsho Shinkeigaku.2004 Jan; 44 (1):7-13.
47. Oliver K. Mohrs, Steffen E.Peresen, Damir E. et al. Diagnosis of patent foramen ovale using contrast-enhanced dynamic MRI: a pilot study.
48. George W. Petty, MD; Bijoy K. Khanderia, MD; Irene eissener, MD; et al. Population-Based Study of the Relationship Between Patent Foramen Ovale and Cerebrovascular Ischemic Events. Mayo Clin Proc. 2006;81(5):602-608.

49. Schwerzmann M, Seiler C, Lipp E, et al. Relation between directly detected patent foramen ovale and ischemic brain lesions in sport divers. Ann Intern Med 2001;134:21-4
50. Bove AA. Risk of decompression sickness with patent foramen ovale. Undersea Hyperb Med 1998;25:175-8
51. Marcuss Schwerzmann, C. Seiler.Recreational scuba diving, patent foramen ovale and their associated risks. Swiss Med Wkly 2001 :131:365-374.
52. Harald Lethen, htD, Frank A. Iachskampf, MD, Rolf Schneider, MD, etal.Frequency of Deep Vein Thrombosis in Patients with Patent Foramen Ovale and Ischemic Stroke or Transient Ischemic Attack. 1997 by Excerpta Medica, Inc.(Am J Cardiol 1997;80: 1066-I 069).
53. Landi G, D'Angelo A, Boccardi E, et al. Venous thromboembolism in acute stroke: prognostic importance of hypercoagulability. Arch Neuml 1992; 49:27Y-283.
54. G. DI Minno,*_ P. M. Mannucci, ** A. Tufano,*et al. The first ambulatory screening on thromboembolism: a multicentre, cross-sectional, observational study on risk factors for venous thromboembolism On behalf of the first ambulatory screening on thromboembolism (fast study group) Journal of Thrombosis and Haemostasis, 3: 1459–1466
55. Schneider B, Zienkiewcz T, Jansen V, et al. Diagnosis of patent foramen ovale by transoesophageal echocardiography and correlation with cerebral and peripheral embolic events. Am J Cardiol 1992; 70:668-772.
56. Pearson AC, Labovitz AJ, Tatineni S, et al. Superiority of transoesophageal echocardiography in detecting cardiac source of embolism in patients with cerebral ischemia of uncertain aetiology. J Am Coll Cardiol 1991; 17:66-72.
57. G. Souteyrand, P. Motreff, J.R.Lusson., et al. Comparison of transthoracic echocardiography using second harmonic imaging, trancranial doppler and transoesophageal echocardiography for the detection of patent foramen ovale in stroke patients. Eur J Echocardiography (2006) 7,147-154.

58. V.Camp.G, Franken P, Melis P, et al. Comparison of transthoracic echocardiography with second harmonic imaging with transoesophageal echocardiography in the detection of right to left shunts. Am J Cardial 2000; 86:1284-7.

59. Daniels C, Weytjens C, Cosyns, et al. Second harmonic transthoracic echocardiography: the new reference screening method for the detection of patent foramen ovale. Eur J Echocardiogr 2004; 5:5449-52.
60. Yoshida M, Goto S, Aikawa M , et al. Detection of right to left shunting through a patent foramen ovale in Japanese patients with ischemic stroke by tranesophageal echocardiography using a standardized valsalva manoeuver. Tokai j Exp Clin Med. 2005 Dec; 30 (4):211-6.
61. Teague SM, Sharma MK. Detection of paradoxical cerebral echo contrast embolization by trancranial doppler ultrasound. Stroke 1991; 22:740-5.
62. Klotzsch C, Janssen G, Berlit P.et al. Transoesophageal echocardiography and contrast-TCD in the detection of a patent foramen ovale: experiences with 111 patients. Neurology 1994;1603-6.
63. Droste DW, Rwisener M, Kemeny V, Dittrich R, et al. Contrast transcranial doppler ultrasound in the detection of right-to-left shunts. Reproducibility, comparison of 2 agents, and distribution of microemboli. Stroke 1999; 30: 1014-8
64. Blersch WK, Draganski BM, Holmer SR, et al. Trancranial duplex sonography in the detection of patent foramen ovale. Radiology 2002; 225:693-9.
65. H. Hara, MD, R. Virmani, MD, E. Iadich, et al. Patent foramen ovale: current pathology, pathophysiology and clinical status. (J Am Coll Cardiol 2005; 46:1768-76).
66. Spencer MP, Moehring MA, Jesurum J, et al. Power M-mode transcranial Doppler for the diagnosis of patent foramen ovale and assessing transcatheter closure. J Neuroimaging 2004; 14:342-9.
67. Moehring MA, Spencer MP. Power M-mode Doppler (PMD) for observing cerebral blood flow and tracing emboli. Ultrasound Med Biol 2002; 28: 49-57.
68. E.Onorato.M.D, G. Melzi. M.D., F. Casilli, M.D. et al. Patent foramen ovale with paradoxical embolism: Mid-term results of transcatheter closure in 256 patients. (J Interven Cardiol2003;16:43-50)

69. S.Klotz, M.D., T.D.T.Tjan, M.D., E. Berendes, M.D., et al. Surgical closure of combined symptomatic patent foramen ovale and atrial septal aneurysm for prevention of recurrent cerebral emboli.
70. K. Nedeltchev, M. Arnold, A. Wahl, et al. Outcome of patients with cryptogenic and patent foramen ovale. J Neurol Neurosurg Psychiatry. 2002; 72:347-350.

71. P. Lechat, Mas JL, Lascault G, et al. Prevalence of patent foramen ovale in patients with stroke. N Engl J Med 1988, 318:1148-52.
72. Hagen PT, Scholz DG, Edwards WD. Incidence and size of patent foramen ovale during the first 10 decades of life: an autopsy study of 965 normal hearts. Mayo Clin Proc 1984; 59:17-20.

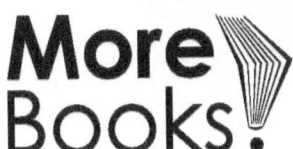 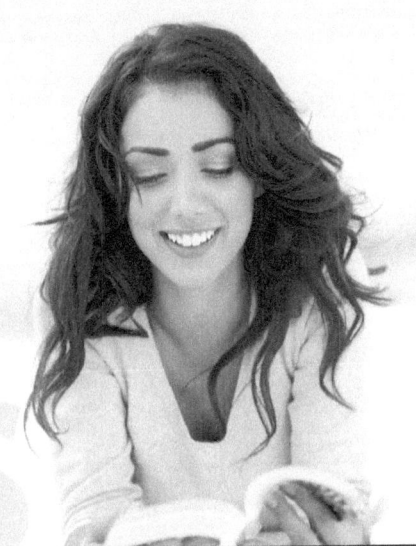

I want morebooks!

Buy your books fast and straightforward online - at one of the world's fastest growing online book stores! Environmentally sound due to Print-on-Demand technologies.

Buy your books online at
www.get-morebooks.com

Kaufen Sie Ihre Bücher schnell und unkompliziert online – auf einer der am schnellsten wachsenden Buchhandelsplattformen weltweit!
Dank Print-On-Demand umwelt- und ressourcenschonend produziert.

Bücher schneller online kaufen
www.morebooks.de

OmniScriptum Marketing DEU GmbH
Heinrich-Böcking-Str. 6-8
D - 66121 Saarbrücken
Telefax: +49 681 93 81 567-9

info@omniscriptum.com
www.omniscriptum.com

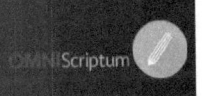

www.ingramcontent.com/pod-product-compliance
Lightning Source LLC
Chambersburg PA
CBHW031544210526
45464CB00003B/1136